VEGETARIAN DIABETIC COOKBOOKS FOR BEGINNERS

The Beginner's Guide to Vegetarian Diabetic Cooking

T. John

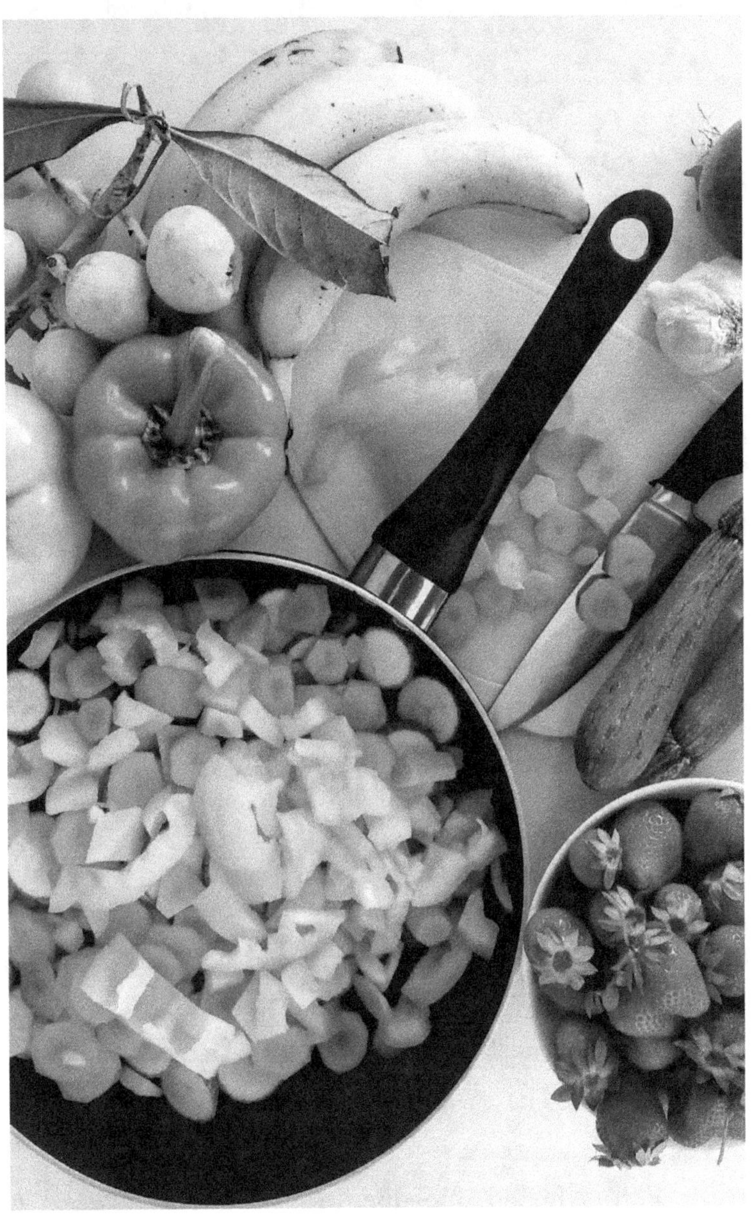

TABLE OF CONTENTS

Chapter 3: Lunch Recipes 39

Chapter 4: Dinner Recipes 61

Chapter 5: Snacks and Appetizers 82

Chapter 6: Desserts 100

Chapter 7: Smoothies 120

INTRODUCTION

Living with diabetes can feel like navigating a labyrinth, but understanding your nutritional needs and exploring new dietary paths can empower you to take control. Today, we delve into the delectable world of vegetarian diets for diabetics, offering insights and beginner-friendly cooking tips to fuel your journey.

Understanding Diabetic Nutrition:

- **Blood Sugar Balance is Key**: Diabetes disrupts your body's ability to regulate blood sugar (glucose). Understanding how different foods impact your glucose levels is crucial. Focus on low-glycemic index (GI) foods that release glucose slowly, preventing spikes and crashes.

- **Fiber is Your Friend**: Fiber slows down digestion, further aiding in stable blood sugar. Load up on non-starchy vegetables, fruits, legumes, and whole grains for a fiber fiesta.

- **Portion Control Matters**: Even healthy foods can impact blood sugar if consumed in excess. Practice mindful eating and use portion control tools like plates and measuring cups.

Benefits of a Vegetarian Diet for Diabetics:

- **Weight Management**: Vegetarian diets tend to be lower in calories and fat, promoting healthy weight management, a crucial factor in diabetes control.
- **Improved Heart Health**: Plant-based diets are rich in fiber, antioxidants, and healthy fats, contributing to lower cholesterol and a healthier heart.
- **Blood Sugar Control**: Studies suggest that well-planned vegetarian diets can improve blood sugar control and insulin sensitivity.

Essential Cooking Tips for Beginners:

- **Embrace Variety**: Explore the vibrant world of plant-based proteins like lentils, beans, tofu, tempeh, and nuts. Experiment with whole grains like quinoa, brown rice, and barley.

- **Spice Up Your Life**: Herbs and spices add flavor without extra calories. Experiment with cumin, turmeric, paprika, and chili powder for an explosion of taste.

- **Master Meatless Mains**: Create satisfying main courses with lentil stews, veggie burgers, tofu scrambles, or stuffed portobello mushrooms.

- **Befriend Vegetables**: Roast, steam, stir-fry, or grill your favorite veggies for a colorful and nutrient-rich side dish.

- **Don't Fear Sweet Treats**: Indulge in moderation with fruits, baked goods sweetened with natural sweeteners like stevia or maple syrup, and dark chocolate.

Embrace the Journey:

Remember, exploring a vegetarian diet is a journey, not a destination. With the right knowledge, planning, and a dash of creativity, you can unlock a world of delicious and nutritious possibilities, empowering you to manage your diabetes with confidence and savor the flavor of good health.

Chapter 1: 30 Day Meal Plan

Week 1:

Day 1:

- Breakfast: Avocado and Tomato Breakfast Sandwich
- Lunch: Lentil and Vegetable Soup
- Dinner: Eggplant Parmesan with Whole Wheat Pasta
- Snack: Guacamole with Veggie Sticks
- Dessert: Sugar-Free Berry Sorbet

Day 2:

- Breakfast: Quinoa Porridge with Berries
- Lunch: Quinoa Salad with Roasted Vegetables
- Dinner: Butternut Squash and Sage Risotto
- Snack: Roasted Chickpeas with Chili and Lime
- Dessert: Chocolate Avocado Mousse

Day 3:

- Breakfast: Spinach and Feta Omelette
- Lunch: Chickpea and Spinach Stuffed Bell Peppers
- Dinner: Cabbage and Lentil Casserole
- Snack: Greek Yogurt and Berry Parfait

- Dessert: Almond Flour Blueberry Muffins

Day 4:

- Breakfast: Chia Seed Pudding with Almond Milk
- Lunch: Greek Salad with Tofu Feta
- Dinner: Portobello Mushroom Steaks with Chimichurri
- Snack: Cucumber and Hummus Bites
- Dessert: Coconut and Mango Chia Pudding

Day 5:

- Breakfast: Whole Grain Pancakes with Sugar-Free Syrup
- Lunch: Cauliflower and Broccoli Rice Bowl
- Dinner: Stuffed Bell Peppers with Quinoa and Black Beans
- Snack: Stuffed Grape Leaves with Quinoa and Herbs
- Dessert: Baked Apples with Cinnamon and Walnuts

Day 6:

- Breakfast: Greek Yogurt Parfait with Nuts and Seeds
- Lunch: Black Bean and Corn Quesadilla

- Dinner: Ratatouille with Herbed Quinoa

- Snack: Edamame and Sea Salt

- Dessert: Pumpkin Pie Smoothie

Day 7:

- Breakfast: Sweet Potato Hash with Poached Eggs

- Lunch: Sweet Potato and Kale Salad

- Dinner: Cauliflower Crust Veggie Pizza

- Snack: Avocado Salsa with Whole Grain Chips

- Dessert: Lemon Poppy Seed Cake with Greek Yogurt Glaze

Week 2:

Day 8:

- Breakfast: Veggie Breakfast Burrito

- Lunch: Spaghetti Squash with Tomato Basil Sauce

- Dinner: Spinach and Artichoke-Stuffed Mushrooms

- Snack: Tomato Basil Bruschetta

- Dessert: Dark Chocolate-Dipped Strawberries

Day 9:

- Breakfast: Blueberry Almond Smoothie Bowl

- Lunch: Mushroom and Asparagus Stir-Fry

- Dinner: Thai Basil Tofu Stir-Fry

- Snack: Spicy Roasted Almonds

- Dessert: Pistachio and Cranberry Energy Bites

Day 10:

- Breakfast: Apple Cinnamon Oatmeal

- Lunch: Caprese Wrap with Balsamic Glaze

- Dinner: Spicy Chickpea and Spinach Curry

- Snack: Caprese Skewers with Balsamic Glaze

- Dessert: Raspberry and Almond Oat Bars

Day 11:

- Breakfast: Broccoli and Cheese Mini Frittatas

- Lunch: Brown Rice and Vegetable Sushi Rolls

- Dinner: Roasted Vegetable and Hummus Wrap

- Snack: Spinach and Artichoke Dip with Whole Grain Pita

- Dessert: Mango and Lime Frozen Yogurt

Day 12:

- Breakfast: Berry and Banana Breakfast Wrap

- Lunch: Thai-inspired Tofu and Vegetable Curry
- Dinner: Zucchini Noodles with Pesto and Cherry Tomatoes
- Snack: Baked Sweet Potato Fries
- Dessert: Vanilla Bean Panna Cotta with Berries

Day 13:

- Breakfast: Zucchini and Mushroom Breakfast Skillet
- Lunch: Spinach and Chickpea Salad with Lemon Vinaigrette
- Dinner: Mexican-Inspired Stuffed Zucchini Boats
- Snack: Berry and Nut Trail Mix
- Dessert: Peach and Almond Crisp

Day 14:

- Breakfast: Protein-Packed Tofu Scramble
- Lunch: Mediterranean Stuffed Portobello Mushrooms
- Dinner: Asparagus and Lemon Risotto
- Snack: Veggie Spring Rolls with Peanut Dipping Sauce

- Dessert: Carrot Cake Bites with Cream Cheese Frosting

Week 3:

Day 15:

- Breakfast: Mango Lime Smoothie
- Lunch: Quinoa and Black Bean Burrito Bowl
- Dinner: Barley and Vegetable Casserole
- Snack: Mini Caprese Salad Skewers
- Dessert: Carrot Cake Bites with Cream Cheese Frosting

Day 16:

- Breakfast: Avocado and Tomato Breakfast Sandwich
- Lunch: Lentil and Vegetable Soup
- Dinner: Eggplant Parmesan with Whole Wheat Pasta
- Snack: Guacamole with Veggie Sticks
- Dessert: Sugar-Free Berry Sorbet

Day 17:

- Breakfast: Quinoa Porridge with Berries
- Lunch: Quinoa Salad with Roasted Vegetables

- Dinner: Butternut Squash and Sage Risotto
- Snack: Roasted Chickpeas with Chili and Lime
- Dessert: Chocolate Avocado Mousse

Day 18:

- Breakfast: Spinach and Feta Omelette
- Lunch: Chickpea and Spinach Stuffed Bell Peppers
- Dinner: Cabbage and Lentil Casserole
- Snack: Greek Yogurt and Berry Parfait
- Dessert: Almond Flour Blueberry Muffins

Day 19:

- Breakfast: Chia Seed Pudding with Almond Milk
- Lunch: Greek Salad with Tofu Feta
- Dinner: Portobello Mushroom Steaks with Chimichurri
- Snack: Cucumber and Hummus Bites
- Dessert: Coconut and Mango Chia Pudding

Day 20:

- Breakfast: Whole Grain Pancakes with Sugar-Free Syrup

- Lunch: Cauliflower and Broccoli Rice Bowl
- Dinner: Stuffed Bell Peppers with Quinoa and Black Beans
- Snack: Stuffed Grape Leaves with Quinoa and Herbs
- Dessert: Baked Apples with Cinnamon and Walnuts

Day 21:

- Breakfast: Greek Yogurt Parfait with Nuts and Seeds
- Lunch: Black Bean and Corn Quesadilla
- Dinner: Ratatouille with Herbed Quinoa
- Snack: Edamame and Sea Salt
- Dessert: Pumpkin Pie Smoothie

Week 4:

Day 22:

- Breakfast: Sweet Potato Hash with Poached Eggs
- Lunch: Sweet Potato and Kale Salad
- Dinner: Cauliflower Crust Veggie Pizza
- Snack: Avocado Salsa with Whole Grain Chips
- Dessert: Lemon Poppy Seed Cake with Greek Yogurt Glaze

Day 23:

- Breakfast: Veggie Breakfast Burrito
- Lunch: Spaghetti Squash with Tomato Basil Sauce
- Dinner: Spinach and Artichoke-Stuffed Mushrooms
- Snack: Tomato Basil Bruschetta
- Dessert: Dark Chocolate-Dipped Strawberries

Day 24:

- Breakfast: Blueberry Almond Smoothie Bowl
- Lunch: Mushroom and Asparagus Stir-Fry
- Dinner: Thai Basil Tofu Stir-Fry
- Snack: Spicy Roasted Almonds
- Dessert: Pistachio and Cranberry Energy Bites

Day 25:

- Breakfast: Apple Cinnamon Oatmeal
- Lunch: Caprese Wrap with Balsamic Glaze
- Dinner: Spicy Chickpea and Spinach Curry
- Snack: Caprese Skewers with Balsamic Glaze
- Dessert: Raspberry and Almond Oat Bars

Day 26:

- Breakfast: Broccoli and Cheese Mini Frittatas
- Lunch: Brown Rice and Vegetable Sushi Rolls
- Dinner: Roasted Vegetable and Hummus Wrap
- Snack: Spinach and Artichoke Dip with Whole Grain Pita
- Dessert: Mango and Lime Frozen Yogurt

Day 27:

- Breakfast: Berry and Banana Breakfast Wrap
- Lunch: Thai-inspired Tofu and Vegetable Curry
- Dinner: Zucchini Noodles with Pesto and Cherry Tomatoes
- Snack: Baked Sweet Potato Fries
- Dessert: Vanilla Bean Panna Cotta with Berries

Day 28:

- Breakfast: Zucchini and Mushroom Breakfast Skillet
- Lunch: Spinach and Chickpea Salad with Lemon Vinaigrette
- Dinner: Mexican-Inspired Stuffed Zucchini Boats
- Snack: Berry and Nut Trail Mix

- Dessert: Peach and Almond Crisp

Day 29:

- Breakfast: Protein-Packed Tofu Scramble
- Lunch: Mediterranean Stuffed Portobello Mushrooms
- Dinner: Asparagus and Lemon Risotto
- Snack: Veggie Spring Rolls with Peanut Dipping Sauce
- Dessert: Carrot Cake Bites with Cream Cheese Frosting

Day 30:

- Breakfast: Mango Lime Smoothie
- Lunch: Quinoa and Black Bean Burrito Bowl
- Dinner: Barley and Vegetable Casserole
- Snack: Mini Caprese Salad Skewers
- Dessert: Carrot Cake Bites with Cream Cheese Frosting

Chapter 2: Breakfast Recipes

This chapter unfolds a tapestry of flavors and nourishing ingredients, presenting you with unique breakfast recipes to kickstart your day. Each recipe is crafted with care, considering both taste and nutritional value

Avocado and Tomato Breakfast Sandwich

Ingredients:

- 1 whole grain English muffin
- 1/2 ripe avocado, sliced
- 1 medium-sized tomato, sliced
- Salt and pepper to taste

Instructions:

1. Toast the English muffin halves.
2. Spread the sliced avocado on one half.
3. Layer the tomato slices on top.
4. Sprinkle with salt and pepper.
5. Top with the other half of the English muffin.

Nutrition Information (per serving):

- Calories: 250
- Protein: 7g
- Carbohydrates: 35g
- Fat: 10g
- Fiber: 8g
- Sugar: 3g
- Portion Size: 1 sandwich

Quinoa Porridge with Berries

Ingredients:

- 1/2 cup quinoa, rinsed
- 1 cup almond milk
- Mixed berries for topping
- Honey or sugar-free sweetener (optional)

Instructions:

1. Cook quinoa in almond milk according to package instructions.
2. Top with mixed berries.
3. Sweeten with honey or a sugar-free sweetener if desired.

Nutrition Information (per serving):

- Calories: 220
- Protein: 8g
- Carbohydrates: 35g
- Fat: 5g
- Fiber: 5g
- Sugar: 4g
- Portion Size: 1 cup

Spinach and Feta Omelette

Ingredients:

- 2 large eggs
- Handful of fresh spinach
- 2 tbsp crumbled feta cheese
- Salt and pepper to taste

Instructions:

1. Whisk eggs and pour into a heated, oiled pan.
2. Add spinach and feta to one side.
3. Fold the omelette in half and cook until eggs are set.

Nutrition Information (per serving):

- Calories: 180
- Protein: 15g
- Carbohydrates: 2g
- Fat: 12g
- Fiber: 1g
- Sugar: 0g
- Portion Size: 1 omelette

Chia Seed Pudding with Almond Milk

Ingredients:

- 2 tbsp chia seeds
- 1 cup unsweetened almond milk
- 1 tsp vanilla extract
- Berries for topping

Instructions:

1. Mix chia seeds, almond milk, and vanilla extract in a bowl.
2. Refrigerate for at least 4 hours or overnight.
3. Top with berries before serving.

Nutrition Information (per serving):

- Calories: 120
- Protein: 4g
- Carbohydrates: 12g
- Fat: 6g
- Fiber: 8g
- Sugar: 1g
- Portion Size: 1/2 cup

Whole Grain Pancakes with Sugar-Free Syrup

Ingredients:

- 1 cup whole grain pancake mix
- 1 cup water
- Sugar-free syrup for topping
- Fresh fruit (optional)

Instructions:

1. Mix pancake mix with water until smooth.
2. Cook pancakes on a griddle or pan.
3. Top with sugar-free syrup and fresh fruit if desired.

Nutrition Information (per serving):

- Calories: 200
- Protein: 5g
- Carbohydrates: 40g
- Fat: 2g
- Fiber: 6g
- Sugar: 2g
- Portion Size: 2 pancakes

Greek Yogurt Parfait with Nuts and Seeds

Ingredients:

- 1 cup Greek yogurt
- 1/4 cup mixed nuts and seeds (almonds, chia seeds, sunflower seeds)
- 1 tbsp honey

Instructions:

1. Layer Greek yogurt in a glass.
2. Add a layer of mixed nuts and seeds.
3. Drizzle with honey.

Nutrition Information (per serving):

- Calories: 280
- Protein: 20g
- Carbohydrates: 15g
- Fat: 18g
- Fiber: 3g
- Sugar: 9g
- Portion Size: 1 cup

Sweet Potato Hash with Poached Eggs

Ingredients:

- 1 medium sweet potato, diced
- 2 eggs
- 1 tbsp olive oil
- Salt and pepper to taste

Instructions:

1. Cook sweet potatoes in olive oil until tender.
2. Poach eggs and place on top of the sweet potatoes.
3. Season with salt and pepper.

Nutrition Information (per serving):

- Calories: 230
- Protein: 10g
- Carbohydrates: 25g
- Fat: 10g
- Fiber: 5g
- Sugar: 6g
- Portion Size: 1 cup

Veggie Breakfast Burrito

Ingredients:

- 1 whole grain tortilla
- 1/2 cup black beans, cooked
- 1/4 cup diced bell peppers
- 2 tbsp salsa

Instructions:

1. Fill the tortilla with black beans, bell peppers, and salsa.
2. Roll into a burrito.

Nutrition Information (per serving):

- Calories: 280
- Protein: 12g
- Carbohydrates: 45g
- Fat: 6g
- Fiber: 10g
- Sugar: 3g
- Portion Size: 1 burrito

Blueberry Almond Smoothie Bowl

Ingredients:

- 1 cup blueberries
- 1/2 banana
- 1/2 cup almond milk
- 1 tbsp almond butter
- Granola for topping

Instructions:

1. Blend blueberries, banana, almond milk, and almond butter.
2. Pour into a bowl and top with granola.

Nutrition Information (per serving):

- Calories: 220
- Protein: 5g
- Carbohydrates: 35g
- Fat: 8g
- Fiber: 7g
- Sugar: 16g
- Portion Size: 1 bowl

Apple Cinnamon Oatmeal

Ingredients:

- 1/2 cup rolled oats
- 1 apple, diced
- 1/2 tsp cinnamon
- 1 cup water or milk

Instructions:

1. Cook oats with diced apples, cinnamon, and water or milk.
2. Stir until creamy and apples are tender.

Nutrition Information (per serving):

- Calories: 200
- Protein: 5g
- Carbohydrates: 40g
- Fat: 3g
- Fiber: 6g
- Sugar: 12g
- Portion Size: 1 cup

Broccoli and Cheese Mini Frittatas

Ingredients:

- 4 large eggs
- 1 cup broccoli florets, steamed and chopped
- 1/2 cup shredded cheddar cheese
- Salt and pepper to taste

Instructions:

1. Preheat the oven to 350°F (175°C).
2. In a bowl, whisk eggs and season with salt and pepper.
3. Stir in chopped broccoli and shredded cheddar.
4. Pour the mixture into greased muffin tins.

5. Bake for 15-20 minutes until set.

Nutrition Information (per serving):

- Calories: 180
- Protein: 12g
- Carbohydrates: 5g
- Fat: 12g
- Fiber: 2g
- Sugar: 1g
- Portion Size: 2 frittatas

Berry and Banana Breakfast Wrap

Ingredients:

- 1 whole grain wrap
- 1/2 cup mixed berries
- 1 banana, sliced
- 2 tbsp Greek yogurt

Instructions:

1. Spread Greek yogurt on the whole grain wrap.
2. Add mixed berries and sliced banana.
3. Roll the wrap and enjoy.

Nutrition Information (per serving):

- Calories: 250
- Protein: 8g
- Carbohydrates: 50g
- Fat: 4g
- Fiber: 8g
- Sugar: 18g
- Portion Size: 1 wrap

Zucchini and Mushroom Breakfast Skillet

Ingredients:

- 1 medium zucchini, diced
- 1 cup mushrooms, sliced
- 2 eggs
- 1 tbsp olive oil
- Salt and pepper to taste

Instructions:

1. Heat olive oil in a skillet.
2. Add diced zucchini and sliced mushrooms.

3. Crack eggs into the skillet and stir until eggs are cooked.

4. Season with salt and pepper.

Nutrition Information (per serving):

- Calories: 200
- Protein: 10g
- Carbohydrates: 8g
- Fat: 15g
- Fiber: 3g
- Sugar: 5g
- Portion Size: 1 cup

Protein-Packed Tofu Scramble

Ingredients:

- 1/2 block firm tofu, crumbled
- 1 cup spinach, chopped
- 1/2 bell pepper, diced
- 1 tsp turmeric
- Salt and pepper to taste

Instructions:

1. In a pan, sauté crumbled tofu with chopped spinach and diced bell pepper.

2. Add turmeric, salt, and pepper. Cook until heated through.

Nutrition Information (per serving):

*   Calories: 180
*   Protein: 15g
*   Carbohydrates: 8g
*   Fat: 10g
*   Fiber: 3g
*   Sugar: 2g
*   Portion Size: 1 cup

Mango Lime Smoothie

Ingredients:

*   1 cup mango chunks
*   Juice of 1 lime
*   1/2 cup Greek yogurt
*   1/2 cup water or coconut water
*   Ice cubes (optional)

Instructions:

1. Blend mango chunks, lime juice, Greek yogurt, and water (or coconut water).

2. Add ice cubes if desired and blend until smooth.

Nutrition Information (per serving):

- Calories: 150
- Protein: 8g
- Carbohydrates: 30g
- Fat: 2g
- Fiber: 3g
- Sugar: 22g
- Portion Size: 1 cup

Chapter 3: Lunch Recipes

These recipes are not just about health; they're about savoring every bite and enjoying a diverse range of flavors. Each dish is crafted with precision, bringing together wholesome ingredients that cater to both your nutritional requirements and culinary desires

Lentil and Vegetable Soup

Ingredients:

- 1 cup green lentils
- 2 carrots, diced
- 1 onion, chopped
- 2 celery stalks, sliced
- 3 cloves garlic, minced
- 1 can diced tomatoes
- 6 cups vegetable broth
- 1 teaspoon cumin
- 1 teaspoon paprika
- Salt and pepper to taste

Instructions:

1. Rinse lentils and set aside.
2. In a large pot, sauté onions and garlic until fragrant.
3. Add carrots, celery, lentils, tomatoes, and vegetable broth.
4. Season with cumin, paprika, salt, and pepper.
5. Simmer for 30-40 minutes until lentils are tender.
6. Serve hot.

Nutrition Information:

- Calories: 250
- Protein: 15g
- Carbohydrates: 40g
- Fat: 2g
- Fiber: 12g
- Sugar: 5g
- Portion size: 1 cup

Quinoa Salad with Roasted Vegetables

Ingredients:

- 1 cup quinoa, cooked

- 1 zucchini, diced
- 1 red bell pepper, sliced
- 1 yellow bell pepper, sliced
- 1 cup cherry tomatoes, halved
- 1/4 cup feta cheese, crumbled
- 2 tablespoons olive oil
- 1 tablespoon balsamic vinegar
- Salt and pepper to taste

Instructions:

1. Preheat oven to 400°F (200°C).
2. Toss zucchini, bell peppers, and cherry tomatoes with olive oil.
3. Roast in the oven for 20 minutes.
4. In a bowl, mix cooked quinoa, roasted vegetables, feta, and balsamic vinegar.
5. Season with salt and pepper.
6. Serve chilled.

Nutrition Information:

- Calories: 280
- Protein: 8g

- Carbohydrates: 35g

- Fat: 12g

- Fiber: 6g

- Sugar: 4g

- Portion size: 1 cup

Chickpea and Spinach Stuffed Bell Peppers

Ingredients:

- 4 bell peppers, halved

- 1 can chickpeas, drained and rinsed

- 2 cups spinach, chopped

- 1 onion, diced

- 2 cloves garlic, minced

- 1 teaspoon cumin

- 1 teaspoon smoked paprika

- 1/2 cup tomato sauce

- 1/2 cup shredded mozzarella cheese (optional)

- Salt and pepper to taste

Instructions:

1. Preheat oven to 375°F (190°C).

2. In a skillet, sauté onions and garlic until soft.

3. Add chickpeas, spinach, cumin, and smoked paprika. Cook until spinach wilts.

4. Stir in tomato sauce and season with salt and pepper.

5. Spoon the mixture into halved bell peppers.

6. Top with mozzarella if desired.

7. Bake for 25-30 minutes.

Nutrition Information:

- Calories: 220
- Protein: 10g
- Carbohydrates: 30g
- Fat: 7g
- Fiber: 8g
- Sugar: 6g
- Portion size: 1 pepper half

Greek Salad with Tofu Feta

Ingredients:

- 2 cups mixed salad greens
- 1 cucumber, sliced
- 1 cup cherry tomatoes, halved

- 1/2 red onion, thinly sliced
- 1/2 cup Kalamata olives, pitted
- 1/2 cup firm tofu, crumbled
- 2 tablespoons olive oil
- 1 tablespoon red wine vinegar
- 1 teaspoon dried oregano
- Salt and pepper to taste

Instructions:

1. In a large bowl, combine salad greens, cucumber, tomatoes, red onion, and olives.
2. In a small bowl, whisk together olive oil, red wine vinegar, oregano, salt, and pepper.
3. Drizzle the dressing over the salad and toss to combine.
4. Sprinkle crumbled tofu on top.
5. Serve chilled.

Nutrition Information:

- Calories: 180
- Protein: 8g
- Carbohydrates: 15g

- Fat: 10g
- Fiber: 5g
- Sugar: 3g
- Portion size: 2 cups

Cauliflower and Broccoli Rice Bowl

Ingredients:

- 2 cups cauliflower rice
- 2 cups broccoli florets
- 1 bell pepper, diced
- 1 carrot, grated
- 2 tablespoons soy sauce
- 1 tablespoon sesame oil
- 1 teaspoon ginger, minced
- 1 clove garlic, minced
- 1 green onion, sliced

Instructions:

1. In a wok or skillet, sauté ginger and garlic in sesame oil.
2. Add cauliflower rice, broccoli, bell pepper, and carrot.

3. Stir-fry until vegetables are tender-crisp.

4. Pour in soy sauce and toss to coat.

5. Garnish with green onions.

6. Serve hot.

Nutrition Information:

- Calories: 160

- Protein: 6g

- Carbohydrates: 20g

- Fat: 8g

- Fiber: 8g

- Sugar: 6g

- Portion size: 1.5 cups

Black Bean and Corn Quesadilla

Ingredients:

- 4 whole wheat tortillas

- 1 can black beans, drained and rinsed

- 1 cup corn kernels

- 1 cup diced bell peppers (any color)

- 1 cup shredded cheddar cheese

- 1 teaspoon cumin

- 1 teaspoon chili powder
- 1/2 cup salsa (for serving)

Instructions:

1. In a bowl, mix black beans, corn, bell peppers, cumin, and chili powder.
2. Place a tortilla on a heated skillet.
3. Spoon the bean mixture onto half of the tortilla.
4. Sprinkle with cheese and fold the tortilla in half.
5. Cook until both sides are golden brown.
6. Repeat for remaining quesadillas.
7. Serve with salsa.

Nutrition Information:

- Calories: 300
- Protein: 14g
- Carbohydrates: 40g
- Fat: 10g
- Fiber: 8g
- Sugar: 3g
- Portion size: 1 quesadilla

Sweet Potato and Kale Salad

Ingredients:

- 2 sweet potatoes, peeled and diced
- 4 cups kale, chopped
- 1/2 cup dried cranberries
- 1/4 cup pumpkin seeds
- 1/4 cup feta cheese, crumbled
- 2 tablespoons olive oil
- 1 tablespoon balsamic vinegar
- Salt and pepper to taste

Instructions:

1. Roast sweet potatoes in the oven until tender.
2. Massage kale with olive oil until slightly wilted.
3. In a large bowl, combine kale, roasted sweet potatoes, cranberries, pumpkin seeds, and feta.
4. Drizzle with balsamic vinegar.
5. Toss to combine.
6. Season with salt and pepper.
7. Serve at room temperature.

Nutrition Information:

- Calories: 280
- Protein: 8g
- Carbohydrates: 35g
- Fat: 12g
- Fiber: 7g
- Sugar: 10g
- Portion size: 2 cups

Spaghetti Squash with Tomato Basil Sauce

Ingredients:

- 1 medium spaghetti squash
- 2 cups cherry tomatoes, halved
- 2 cloves garlic, minced
- 1/4 cup fresh basil, chopped
- 2 tablespoons olive oil
- Salt and pepper to taste
- Grated Parmesan cheese (optional)

Instructions:

1. Preheat oven to 400°F (200°C).

2. Cut spaghetti squash in half lengthwise and remove seeds.

3. Place squash halves on a baking sheet, cut side down.

4. Roast for 40-45 minutes or until fork-tender.

5. In a skillet, sauté garlic in olive oil until fragrant.

6. Add cherry tomatoes and cook until softened.

7. Use a fork to shred the spaghetti squash into "noodles."

8. Toss the squash with the tomato-basil sauce.

9. Season with salt and pepper.

10. Top with Parmesan if desired.

Nutrition Information:

- Calories: 220
- Protein: 5g
- Carbohydrates: 30g
- Fat: 10g
- Fiber: 7g
- Sugar: 10g
- Portion size: 2 cups

Mushroom and Asparagus Stir-Fry

Ingredients:

- 2 cups asparagus, trimmed and cut into 2-inch pieces
- 2 cups mushrooms, sliced
- 1 red bell pepper, thinly sliced
- 2 tablespoons soy sauce
- 1 tablespoon sesame oil
- 1 tablespoon rice vinegar
- 1 teaspoon ginger, grated
- 2 cloves garlic, minced
- 1 tablespoon sesame seeds (for garnish)

Instructions:

1. In a wok or skillet, heat sesame oil.
2. Sauté ginger and garlic until aromatic.
3. Add mushrooms, asparagus, and bell pepper.
4. Stir-fry until vegetables are tender-crisp.
5. Mix in soy sauce and rice vinegar.
6. Garnish with sesame seeds.
7. Serve over brown rice or quinoa.

Nutrition Information:

- Calories: 150
- Protein: 6g
- Carbohydrates: 15g
- Fat: 8g
- Fiber: 5g
- Sugar: 5g
- Portion size: 1.5 cups

Caprese Wrap with Balsamic Glaze

Ingredients:

- 4 whole wheat wraps
- 2 large tomatoes, sliced
- 1 cup fresh mozzarella, sliced
- 1 cup fresh basil leaves
- 2 tablespoons balsamic glaze
- Salt and pepper to taste

Instructions:

1. Lay out the whole wheat wraps.
2. Layer each wrap with tomato slices, mozzarella, and fresh basil.

3. Drizzle with balsamic glaze.

4. Season with salt and pepper.

5. Wrap tightly and slice in half.

6. Serve chilled.

Nutrition Information:

- Calories: 320

- Protein: 15g

- Carbohydrates: 35g

- Fat: 15g

- Fiber: 6g

- Sugar: 8g

- Portion size: 1 wrap

Brown Rice and Vegetable Sushi Rolls

Ingredients:

- 2 cups brown rice, cooked

- 4 nori seaweed sheets

- 1 cucumber, julienned

- 1 avocado, sliced

- 1 carrot, julienned

- 1/2 cup pickled ginger

- Soy sauce for dipping

- Wasabi and sesame seeds for garnish

Instructions:

1. Place a nori sheet on a bamboo sushi mat.

2. Spread a thin layer of brown rice over the nori, leaving a small border.

3. Arrange cucumber, avocado, and carrot along the center.

4. Roll the sushi tightly, using the bamboo mat as a guide.

5. Seal the edge with a dab of water.

6. Slice into bite-sized pieces.

7. Serve with pickled ginger, soy sauce, wasabi, and sprinkle with sesame seeds.

Nutrition Information:

- Calories: 250

- Protein: 6g

- Carbohydrates: 45g

- Fat: 6g

- Fiber: 8g
- Sugar: 2g
- Portion size: 8 pieces

Thai-inspired Tofu and Vegetable Curry

Ingredients:

- 1 block firm tofu, cubed
- 2 cups mixed vegetables (broccoli, bell peppers, snap peas)
- 1 can coconut milk
- 2 tablespoons red curry paste
- 1 tablespoon soy sauce
- 1 tablespoon brown sugar
- 1 tablespoon lime juice
- Fresh cilantro for garnish
- Cooked jasmine rice (optional)

Instructions:

1. In a wok or skillet, sauté tofu until golden brown.
2. Add mixed vegetables and stir-fry until crisp-tender.

3. In a bowl, mix coconut milk, red curry paste, soy sauce, brown sugar, and lime juice.

4. Pour the curry sauce over the tofu and vegetables.

5. Simmer for 10-15 minutes.

6. Garnish with fresh cilantro.

7. Serve over jasmine rice if desired.

Nutrition Information:

- Calories: 300

- Protein: 12g

- Carbohydrates: 20g

- Fat: 18g

- Fiber: 6g

- Sugar: 8g

- Portion size: 1.5 cups curry (without rice)

Spinach and Chickpea Salad with Lemon Vinaigrette

Ingredients:

- 4 cups fresh spinach

- 1 can chickpeas, drained and rinsed

- 1 cup cherry tomatoes, halved

- 1/2 red onion, thinly sliced
- 1/4 cup feta cheese, crumbled
- 1/4 cup pine nuts, toasted
- 2 tablespoons olive oil
- 1 tablespoon lemon juice
- 1 teaspoon Dijon mustard
- Salt and pepper to taste

Instructions:

1. In a large bowl, combine fresh spinach, chickpeas, cherry tomatoes, red onion, feta, and pine nuts.
2. In a small bowl, whisk together olive oil, lemon juice, Dijon mustard, salt, and pepper.
3. Drizzle the lemon vinaigrette over the salad.
4. Toss gently to coat.
5. Serve immediately.

Nutrition Information:

- Calories: 280
- Protein: 10g
- Carbohydrates: 25g
- Fat: 16g

- Fiber: 7g
- Sugar: 5g
- Portion size: 2 cups

Mediterranean Stuffed Portobello Mushrooms

Ingredients:

- 4 large Portobello mushrooms
- 1 cup quinoa, cooked
- 1 cup cherry tomatoes, diced
- 1/2 cup Kalamata olives, chopped
- 1/4 cup red onion, finely diced
- 2 cloves garlic, minced
- 1/4 cup feta cheese, crumbled
- 2 tablespoons balsamic glaze
- Fresh basil for garnish

Instructions:

1. Preheat oven to 375°F (190°C).
2. Remove the stems from the Portobello mushrooms and clean the caps.

3. In a bowl, mix cooked quinoa, cherry tomatoes, olives, red onion, garlic, and feta.

4. Stuff each Portobello cap with the quinoa mixture.

5. Bake for 20-25 minutes until mushrooms are tender.

6. Drizzle with balsamic glaze.

7. Garnish with fresh basil.

Nutrition Information:

- Calories: 230
- Protein: 10g
- Carbohydrates: 35g
- Fat: 8g
- Fiber: 7g
- Sugar: 5g
- Portion size: 1 mushroom

Quinoa and Black Bean Burrito Bowl

Ingredients:

- 1 cup quinoa, cooked
- 1 can black beans, drained and rinsed
- 1 cup corn kernels
- 1 cup cherry tomatoes, halved

- 1 avocado, sliced
- 1/4 cup cilantro, chopped
- Lime wedges for serving
- Salsa and Greek yogurt for topping

Instructions:

1. In a bowl, assemble quinoa, black beans, corn, cherry tomatoes, avocado, and cilantro.
2. Squeeze lime wedges over the bowl.
3. Top with salsa and Greek yogurt.
4. Mix well before serving.

Nutrition Information:

- Calories: 320
- Protein: 12g
- Carbohydrates: 45g
- Fat: 10g
- Fiber: 10g
- Sugar: 5g
- Portion size: 2 cups

Chapter 4: Dinner Recipes

This chapter unfolds with a collection of dinner recipes carefully crafted to balance taste and nutritional value. From Eggplant Parmesan to Mexican-Inspired Stuffed Zucchini Boats, each dish presents a delectable fusion of ingredients.

Eggplant Parmesan with Whole Wheat Pasta

Ingredients:

- 1 large eggplant, sliced
- 1 cup whole wheat pasta
- 2 cups marinara sauce
- 1 cup shredded mozzarella cheese
- 1/2 cup grated Parmesan cheese
- Fresh basil leaves for garnish

Instructions:

1. Preheat the oven to 375°F (190°C).
2. Salt the eggplant slices and let them sit for 30 minutes to draw out excess moisture.

3. Rinse the eggplant slices and pat them dry.

4. In a baking dish, layer marinara sauce, eggplant slices, and cheeses.

5. Repeat the layers, finishing with a cheese layer on top.

6. Bake for 30-35 minutes until golden and bubbly.

7. Cook whole wheat pasta according to package instructions.

8. Serve the eggplant Parmesan over whole wheat pasta.

Nutrition Information (per serving):

- Calories: 350
- Protein: 15g
- Carbohydrates: 40g
- Fat: 15g
- Fiber: 8g
- Sugar: 10g
- Portion Size: 1 serving

Butternut Squash and Sage Risotto

Ingredients:

- 1 cup Arborio rice
- 2 cups butternut squash, diced
- 1 onion, finely chopped
- 4 cups vegetable broth, heated
- 1/2 cup dry white wine
- 2 tbsp olive oil
- Fresh sage leaves for garnish

Instructions:

1. Sauté onions in olive oil until translucent.
2. Add Arborio rice and cook for 2 minutes.
3. Pour in the white wine and cook until absorbed.
4. Gradually add hot vegetable broth, stirring continuously.
5. Stir in diced butternut squash and cook until rice is creamy and squash is tender.
6. Garnish with fresh sage leaves before serving.

Nutrition Information (per serving):

- Calories: 300

- Protein: 6g

- Carbohydrates: 55g

- Fat: 5g

- Fiber: 5g

- Sugar: 3g

- Portion Size: 1 serving

Cabbage and Lentil Casserole

Ingredients:

- 2 cups green lentils, cooked

- 1 small cabbage, shredded

- 1 onion, diced

- 3 cloves garlic, minced

- 1 can diced tomatoes

- 1 tsp cumin

- 1 tsp paprika

- Salt and pepper to taste

Instructions:

1. Sauté onions and garlic until fragrant.

2. Add shredded cabbage and cook until wilted.

3. Stir in cooked lentils, diced tomatoes, cumin, paprika, salt, and pepper.

4. Transfer to a casserole dish and bake at 350°F (180°C) for 25-30 minutes.

Nutrition Information (per serving):

- Calories: 250

- Protein: 18g

- Carbohydrates: 40g

- Fat: 2g

- Fiber: 15g

- Sugar: 8g

- Portion Size: 1 serving

Portobello Mushroom Steaks with Chimichurri

Ingredients:

- 4 large portobello mushrooms, stems removed

- 1/4 cup olive oil

- 2 tbsp red wine vinegar

- 3 cloves garlic, minced

- 1/4 cup fresh parsley, chopped

- Salt and pepper to taste

Instructions:

1. Preheat the grill or grill pan.
2. Whisk together olive oil, red wine vinegar, garlic, parsley, salt, and pepper to create the chimichurri sauce.
3. Brush portobello mushrooms with the chimichurri sauce.
4. Grill mushrooms for 5-7 minutes per side.
5. Drizzle with additional chimichurri before serving.

Nutrition Information (per serving):

- Calories: 180
- Protein: 5g
- Carbohydrates: 8g
- Fat: 15g
- Fiber: 3g
- Sugar: 3g
- Portion Size: 1 serving

Stuffed Bell Peppers with Quinoa and Black Beans

Ingredients:

- 4 large bell peppers, halved and seeds removed
- 1 cup quinoa, cooked
- 1 can black beans, drained and rinsed
- 1 cup corn kernels
- 1 cup diced tomatoes
- 1 tsp cumin
- 1 tsp chili powder
- 1/2 cup shredded cheddar cheese

Instructions:

1. Preheat the oven to 375°F (190°C).
2. In a bowl, mix cooked quinoa, black beans, corn, tomatoes, cumin, and chili powder.
3. Stuff bell pepper halves with the quinoa mixture.
4. Top with shredded cheddar cheese.
5. Bake for 20-25 minutes until peppers are tender.

Nutrition Information (per serving):

- Calories: 280

- Protein: 12g

- Carbohydrates: 45g

- Fat: 7g

- Fiber: 9g

- Sugar: 5g

- Portion Size: 1 serving

Ratatouille with Herbed Quinoa

Ingredients:

- 1 eggplant, diced

- 1 zucchini, sliced

- 1 yellow squash, sliced

- 1 bell pepper, diced

- 1 onion, sliced

- 2 cloves garlic, minced

- 1 can crushed tomatoes

- 1 tsp dried thyme

- 1 tsp dried rosemary

- 1 cup quinoa, cooked

- Fresh basil for garnish

Instructions:

1. Sauté onion and garlic until softened.
2. Add eggplant, zucchini, yellow squash, bell pepper, crushed tomatoes, thyme, and rosemary.
3. Simmer until vegetables are tender.
4. Serve over a bed of herbed quinoa.
5. Garnish with fresh basil.

Nutrition Information (per serving):

- Calories: 320
- Protein: 10g
- Carbohydrates: 60g
- Fat: 5g
- Fiber: 12g
- Sugar: 10g
- Portion Size: 1 serving

Cauliflower Crust Veggie Pizza

Ingredients:

- 1 cauliflower head, grated
- 1 cup mozzarella cheese, shredded
- 1 egg

- 1 tsp dried oregano
- 1/2 cup tomato sauce
- Assorted veggies (bell peppers, tomatoes, olives)
- Fresh basil for garnish

Instructions:

1. Mix grated cauliflower, mozzarella, egg, and oregano to form the pizza crust.
2. Press the mixture onto a lined baking sheet and bake at 425°F (220°C) for 15 minutes.
3. Spread tomato sauce over the crust and top with veggies.
4. Bake for an additional 10-12 minutes.
5. Garnish with fresh basil before serving.

Nutrition Information (per serving):

- Calories: 220
- Protein: 15g
- Carbohydrates: 20g
- Fat: 10g
- Fiber: 8g
- Sugar: 5g

- Portion Size: 1 serving

Spinach and Artichoke-Stuffed Mushrooms

Ingredients:

- 16 large mushrooms, stems removed
- 1 cup frozen spinach, thawed and drained
- 1 cup artichoke hearts, chopped
- 1/2 cup cream cheese
- 1/4 cup grated Parmesan cheese
- 2 cloves garlic, minced
- Salt and pepper to taste

Instructions:

1. Preheat the oven to 375°F (190°C).
2. In a bowl, mix spinach, artichoke hearts, cream cheese, Parmesan, garlic, salt, and pepper.
3. Stuff mushroom caps with the mixture.
4. Bake for 15-20 minutes until mushrooms are tender.

Nutrition Information (per serving):

- Calories: 150

- Protein: 8g

- Carbohydrates: 10g

- Fat: 9g

- Fiber: 3g

- Sugar: 2g

- Portion Size: 1 serving

Thai Basil Tofu Stir-Fry

Ingredients:

- 1 block extra-firm tofu, pressed and cubed

- 2 cups broccoli florets

- 1 bell pepper, sliced

- 1 carrot, julienned

- 2 tbsp soy sauce

- 1 tbsp hoisin sauce

- 1 tbsp sesame oil

- 1 tsp fresh ginger, minced

- Fresh basil leaves for garnish

Instructions:

1. Sauté tofu in sesame oil until golden brown.

2. Add broccoli, bell pepper, carrot, soy sauce, hoisin sauce, and ginger.

3. Stir-fry until veggies are tender-crisp.

4. Garnish with fresh basil before serving.

Nutrition Information (per serving):

- Calories: 280

- Protein: 18g

- Carbohydrates: 20g

- Fat: 15g

- Fiber: 6g

- Sugar: 8g

- Portion Size: 1 serving

Spicy Chickpea and Spinach Curry

Ingredients:

- 2 cans chickpeas, drained and rinsed

- 1 onion, finely chopped

- 3 cloves garlic, minced

- 1 tsp cumin

- 1 tsp coriander

- 1 tsp turmeric

- 1/2 tsp cayenne pepper
- 1 can diced tomatoes
- 2 cups fresh spinach
- 1/2 cup coconut milk

Instructions:

1. Sauté onions and garlic until softened.
2. Add chickpeas, cumin, coriander, turmeric, and cayenne pepper.
3. Stir in diced tomatoes and coconut milk.
4. Simmer for 15-20 minutes.
5. Add fresh spinach and cook until wilted.

Nutrition Information (per serving):

- Calories: 320
- Protein: 14g
- Carbohydrates: 45g
- Fat: 10g
- Fiber: 12g
- Sugar: 8g
- Portion Size: 1 serving

Roasted Vegetable and Hummus Wrap

Ingredients:

- 1 whole wheat wrap
- 1/2 cup hummus
- Assorted roasted vegetables (zucchini, bell peppers, cherry tomatoes)
- Fresh parsley for garnish

Instructions:

1. Spread hummus over the whole wheat wrap.
2. Arrange roasted vegetables on top.
3. Roll the wrap and garnish with fresh parsley.

Nutrition Information (per serving):

- Calories: 250
- Protein: 10g
- Carbohydrates: 35g
- Fat: 8g
- Fiber: 8g
- Sugar: 5g
- Portion Size: 1 serving

Zucchini Noodles with Pesto and Cherry Tomatoes

Ingredients:

- 2 large zucchinis, spiralized
- 1 cup cherry tomatoes, halved
- 1/2 cup fresh basil leaves
- 1/4 cup pine nuts
- 1/4 cup grated Parmesan cheese
- 2 cloves garlic
- 1/3 cup extra virgin olive oil
- Salt and pepper to taste

Instructions:

1. In a blender, combine basil, pine nuts, Parmesan, garlic, salt, and pepper.
2. Gradually add olive oil and blend until smooth.
3. Toss zucchini noodles with pesto and cherry tomatoes.
4. Serve immediately.

Nutrition Information (per serving):

- Calories: 220

- Protein: 6g

- Carbohydrates: 10g

- Fat: 18g

- Fiber: 4g

- Sugar: 5g

- Portion Size: 1 serving

Mexican-Inspired Stuffed Zucchini Boats

Ingredients:

- 4 large zucchini, halved

- 1 cup black beans, cooked

- 1 cup corn kernels

- 1 cup diced tomatoes

- 1 tsp cumin

- 1 tsp chili powder

- 1/2 cup shredded Monterey Jack cheese

- Fresh cilantro for garnish

Instructions:

1. Preheat the oven to 375°F (190°C).

2. Scoop out the center of each zucchini half to create a boat.

3. In a bowl, mix black beans, corn, tomatoes, cumin, and chili powder.

4. Stuff each zucchini boat with the mixture.

5. Top with shredded cheese and bake for 20-25 minutes.

6. Garnish with fresh cilantro before serving.

Nutrition Information (per serving):

- Calories: 280
- Protein: 12g
- Carbohydrates: 40g
- Fat: 8g
- Fiber: 10g
- Sugar: 8g
- Portion Size: 1 serving

Asparagus and Lemon Risotto

Ingredients:

- 1 cup Arborio rice
- 1 bunch asparagus, trimmed and cut into pieces

- 1 onion, finely chopped

- 4 cups vegetable broth, heated

- 1/2 cup dry white wine

- Zest and juice of 1 lemon

- 2 tbsp olive oil

- Fresh parsley for garnish

Instructions:

1. Sauté onions in olive oil until translucent.

2. Add Arborio rice and cook for 2 minutes.

3. Pour in the white wine and cook until absorbed.

4. Gradually add hot vegetable broth, stirring continuously.

5. Stir in asparagus, lemon zest, and lemon juice.

6. Cook until rice is creamy and asparagus is tender.

7. Garnish with fresh parsley before serving.

Nutrition Information (per serving):

- Calories: 300

- Protein: 6g

- Carbohydrates: 55g

- Fat: 5g

- Fiber: 5g

- Sugar: 3g

- Portion Size: 1 serving

Barley and Vegetable Casserole

Ingredients:

- 1 cup pearl barley, cooked

- 2 cups mixed vegetables (carrots, peas, corn)

- 1 onion, diced

- 2 cloves garlic, minced

- 1 can diced tomatoes

- 1 tsp dried thyme

- 1 tsp dried rosemary

- 1/2 cup vegetable broth

- Salt and pepper to taste

Instructions:

1. Sauté onions and garlic until softened.

2. Add mixed vegetables and cook until slightly tender.

3. Stir in cooked barley, diced tomatoes, thyme, rosemary, vegetable broth, salt, and pepper.

4. Transfer to a casserole dish and bake at 350°F (180°C) for 25-30 minutes.

Nutrition Information (per serving):

- Calories: 250
- Protein: 10g
- Carbohydrates: 50g
- Fat: 2g
- Fiber: 10g
- Sugar: 5g
- Portion Size: 1 serving

Chapter 5: Snacks and Appetizers

These recipes not only cater to your taste buds but also prioritize health, ensuring each bite is a burst of nourishment. Whether you're hosting a gathering or simply treating yourself, these creations are designed to satisfy cravings without compromising your commitment to a vegetarian diabetic diet.

Guacamole with Veggie Sticks

Ingredients:

- 2 ripe avocados
- 1 medium tomato, diced
- 1/4 cup red onion, finely chopped
- 1 clove garlic, minced
- 1 lime, juiced
- Salt and pepper to taste
- Assorted veggie sticks (carrots, bell peppers, cucumber)

Instructions:

1. Mash the avocados in a bowl.

2. Add diced tomatoes, chopped red onion, minced garlic, and lime juice.

3. Season with salt and pepper, then mix until well combined.

4. Serve with a variety of veggie sticks for dipping.

Nutrition Information:

- Calories: 120
- Protein: 2g
- Carbohydrates: 8g
- Fat: 10g
- Fiber: 5g
- Sugar: 1g
- Portion size: 2 tablespoons guacamole with veggie sticks.

Roasted Chickpeas with Chili and Lime

Ingredients:

- 1 can (15 oz) chickpeas, drained and rinsed
- 1 tablespoon olive oil
- 1 teaspoon chili powder

- Zest of 1 lime

- Salt to taste

Instructions:

1. Preheat the oven to 400°F (200°C).

2. Toss chickpeas with olive oil, chili powder, lime zest, and salt.

3. Spread on a baking sheet and roast for 20-25 minutes until crispy.

Nutrition Information:

- Calories: 160

- Protein: 5g

- Carbohydrates: 22g

- Fat: 7g

- Fiber: 6g

- Sugar: 1g

- Portion size: 1/2 cup.

Greek Yogurt and Berry Parfait

Ingredients:

- 1 cup Greek yogurt

- 1/2 cup mixed berries (strawberries, blueberries, raspberries)
- 2 tablespoons honey
- Granola for topping

Instructions:

1. In a glass, layer Greek yogurt, mixed berries, and drizzle with honey.
2. Repeat the layers.
3. Top with granola before serving.

Nutrition Information:

- Calories: 250
- Protein: 15g
- Carbohydrates: 35g
- Fat: 6g
- Fiber: 4g
- Sugar: 20g
- Portion size: 1 serving.

Cucumber and Hummus Bites

Ingredients:

- 1 cucumber, sliced
- 1/2 cup hummus
- Cherry tomatoes, halved
- Fresh parsley for garnish

Instructions:

1. Slice cucumber into rounds.
2. Spoon a small amount of hummus onto each cucumber slice.
3. Top with a halved cherry tomato and garnish with fresh parsley.

Nutrition Information:

- Calories: 70
- Protein: 3g
- Carbohydrates: 8g
- Fat: 3g
- Fiber: 2g
- Sugar: 1g
- Portion size: 4 cucumber and hummus bites.

Stuffed Grape Leaves with Quinoa and Herbs

Ingredients:

- 1 cup quinoa, cooked
- Grape leaves (canned or fresh, blanched)
- 1/4 cup fresh dill, chopped
- 1/4 cup fresh mint, chopped
- Lemon wedges for serving

Instructions:

1. Mix cooked quinoa, chopped dill, and mint in a bowl.
2. Place a spoonful of the quinoa mixture onto each grape leaf.
3. Roll tightly and serve with lemon wedges.

Nutrition Information:

- Calories: 120
- Protein: 4g
- Carbohydrates: 20g
- Fat: 2g
- Fiber: 3g
- Sugar: 0g

- Portion size: 3 stuffed grape leaves.

Edamame and Sea Salt

Ingredients:

- 1 cup edamame, steamed
- Sea salt to taste

Instructions:

1. Steam the edamame according to package instructions.
2. Sprinkle with sea salt while still warm.
3. Serve as a nutritious and satisfying snack.

Nutrition Information:

- Calories: 120
- Protein: 11g
- Carbohydrates: 9g
- Fat: 4g
- Fiber: 5g
- Sugar: 2g
- Portion size: 1 cup.

Avocado Salsa with Whole Grain Chips

Ingredients:

- 2 avocados, diced
- 1 cup cherry tomatoes, halved
- 1/4 cup red onion, finely chopped
- 1 jalapeño, seeded and minced
- 2 tablespoons fresh cilantro, chopped
- Lime juice, to taste
- Whole grain tortilla chips

Instructions:

1. In a bowl, combine diced avocados, cherry tomatoes, red onion, jalapeño, and cilantro.
2. Squeeze lime juice over the mixture and gently toss.
3. Serve with whole grain tortilla chips.

Nutrition Information:

- Calories: 160
- Protein: 3g
- Carbohydrates: 18g
- Fat: 10g

- Fiber: 6g

- Sugar: 2g

- Portion size: 1/2 cup salsa with chips.

Tomato Basil Bruschetta

Ingredients:

- 4 ripe tomatoes, diced

- 1/4 cup fresh basil, chopped

- 2 cloves garlic, minced

- 2 tablespoons extra-virgin olive oil

- Salt and pepper to taste

- Baguette slices, toasted

Instructions:

1. In a bowl, combine diced tomatoes, chopped basil, minced garlic, and olive oil.

2. Season with salt and pepper, then mix well.

3. Spoon the mixture onto toasted baguette slices.

Nutrition Information:

- Calories: 140

- Protein: 3g

- Carbohydrates: 18g

- Fat: 7g

- Fiber: 2g

- Sugar: 2g

- Portion size: 2 slices of bruschetta.

Spicy Roasted Almonds

Ingredients:

- 1 cup almonds

- 1 tablespoon olive oil

- 1 teaspoon chili powder

- 1/2 teaspoon cayenne pepper

- Salt to taste

Instructions:

1. Preheat the oven to 350°F (175°C).

2. Toss almonds with olive oil, chili powder, cayenne pepper, and salt.

3. Spread on a baking sheet and roast for 10-12 minutes, stirring halfway.

Nutrition Information:

- Calories: 180
- Protein: 6g
- Carbohydrates: 6g
- Fat: 15g
- Fiber: 4g
- Sugar: 1g
- Portion size: 1/4 cup.

Caprese Skewers with Balsamic Glaze

Ingredients:

- Cherry tomatoes
- Fresh mozzarella balls
- Fresh basil leaves
- Balsamic glaze

Instructions:

1. Thread a cherry tomato, mozzarella ball, and basil leaf onto each skewer.
2. Arrange on a serving platter and drizzle with balsamic glaze.

Nutrition Information:

- Calories: 90
- Protein: 5g
- Carbohydrates: 2g
- Fat: 7g
- Fiber: 1g
- Sugar: 1g
- Portion size: 3 skewers.

Spinach and Artichoke Dip with Whole Grain Pita

Ingredients:

- 2 cups fresh spinach, chopped
- 1 can (14 oz) artichoke hearts, drained and chopped
- 1 cup Greek yogurt
- 1 cup shredded mozzarella
- 1/4 cup grated Parmesan
- 1 clove garlic, minced
- Whole grain pita, cut into triangles for dipping

Instructions:

1. In a bowl, mix chopped spinach, artichoke hearts, Greek yogurt, mozzarella, Parmesan, and minced garlic.

2. Transfer to a baking dish and bake at 375°F (190°C) for 20 minutes or until bubbly.

3. Serve with whole grain pita triangles.

Nutrition Information:

*   Calories: 180
*   Protein: 12g
*   Carbohydrates: 10g
*   Fat: 10g
*   Fiber: 3g
*   Sugar: 2g
*   Portion size: 1/4 cup dip with pita.

Baked Sweet Potato Fries

Ingredients:

*   2 sweet potatoes, cut into fries
*   2 tablespoons olive oil
*   1 teaspoon paprika

- 1/2 teaspoon garlic powder

- Salt and pepper to taste

Instructions:

1. Preheat the oven to 425°F (220°C).

2. Toss sweet potato fries with olive oil, paprika, garlic powder, salt, and pepper.

3. Spread on a baking sheet and bake for 25-30 minutes, turning halfway.

Nutrition Information:

- Calories: 150

- Protein: 2g

- Carbohydrates: 26g

- Fat: 5g

- Fiber: 4g

- Sugar: 5g

- Portion size: 1 cup.

Berry and Nut Trail Mix

Ingredients:

- 1/2 cup almonds

- 1/2 cup walnuts
- 1/2 cup dried cranberries
- 1/4 cup dark chocolate chips
- 1/4 cup pumpkin seeds

Instructions:

1. Mix almonds, walnuts, dried cranberries, dark chocolate chips, and pumpkin seeds in a bowl.
2. Portion into small snack-sized bags for convenient grab-and-go.

Nutrition Information:

- Calories: 200
- Protein: 5g
- Carbohydrates: 15g
- Fat: 15g
- Fiber: 3g
- Sugar: 8g
- Portion size: 1/4 cup.

Veggie Spring Rolls with Peanut Dipping Sauce

Ingredients:

- Rice paper wrappers
- 1 cup shredded cabbage
- 1 cup julienned carrots
- 1 cucumber, julienned
- Fresh mint leaves
- Fresh cilantro leaves
- 1/4 cup peanuts, chopped

Instructions:

1. Soak rice paper wrappers in warm water until pliable.
2. Place a small amount of shredded cabbage, carrots, cucumber, mint, and cilantro on each wrapper.
3. Roll tightly, folding in the sides, and serve with peanut dipping sauce.

Nutrition Information:

- Calories: 180
- Protein: 5g
- Carbohydrates: 30g

- Fat: 5g

- Fiber: 4g

- Sugar: 4g

- Portion size: 2 spring rolls with sauce.

Mini Caprese Salad Skewers

Ingredients:

- Cherry tomatoes

- Fresh mozzarella balls

- Fresh basil leaves

- Balsamic glaze

Instructions:

1. Thread a cherry tomato, mozzarella ball, and basil leaf onto each skewer.

2. Arrange on a serving platter and drizzle with balsamic glaze.

Nutrition Information:

- Calories: 100

- Protein: 7g

- Carbohydrates: 2g

- Fat: 7g
- Fiber: 1g
- Sugar: 1g
- Portion size: 3 skewers.

Chapter 6: Desserts

These recipes not only satisfy your sweet tooth but also consider the nutritional needs for those managing diabetes. Enjoy the goodness of natural sweetness, innovative flavors, and satisfying textures without compromising on your well-being.

Sugar-Free Berry Sorbet

Ingredients:

- 2 cups mixed berries (strawberries, blueberries, raspberries)
- 1 tablespoon lemon juice
- 1/4 cup sugar substitute
- 1/2 cup water

Instructions:

1. Combine berries, lemon juice, sugar substitute, and water in a blender.
2. Blend until smooth.
3. Pour the mixture into a shallow dish and freeze for at least 4 hours, stirring every hour.

4. Scoop into bowls, and savor the refreshing sweetness.

Nutrition Information:

- Calories: 60
- Protein: 1g
- Carbohydrates: 15g
- Fat: 0g
- Fiber: 4g
- Sugar: 8g
- Portion Size: 1/2 cup

Chocolate Avocado Mousse

Ingredients:

- 2 ripe avocados
- 1/4 cup unsweetened cocoa powder
- 1/4 cup sugar substitute
- 1 teaspoon vanilla extract
- 1/4 cup almond milk

Instructions:

1. Blend avocados, cocoa powder, sugar substitute, vanilla extract, and almond milk until smooth.
2. Chill in the refrigerator for at least 2 hours.
3. Serve in small bowls for a rich, chocolatey treat.

Nutrition Information:

- Calories: 120
- Protein: 2g
- Carbohydrates: 10g
- Fat: 9g
- Fiber: 5g
- Sugar: 1g
- Portion Size: 1/4 cup

Almond Flour Blueberry Muffins

Ingredients:

- 1 1/2 cups almond flour
- 1/2 teaspoon baking soda
- 1/4 teaspoon salt
- 1/4 cup coconut oil, melted
- 3 tablespoons sugar substitute

- 2 large eggs
- 1 teaspoon vanilla extract
- 1 cup fresh blueberries

Instructions:

1. Preheat the oven to 350°F (175°C) and line a muffin tin with paper liners.
2. In a bowl, combine almond flour, baking soda, and salt.
3. In another bowl, whisk together melted coconut oil, sugar substitute, eggs, and vanilla extract.
4. Mix wet and dry ingredients, then fold in blueberries.
5. Spoon the batter into muffin cups and bake for 20-25 minutes.

Nutrition Information:

- Calories: 150
- Protein: 5g
- Carbohydrates: 8g
- Fat: 12g
- Fiber: 3g
- Sugar: 2g

- Portion Size: 1 muffin

Coconut and Mango Chia Pudding

Ingredients:

- 1/4 cup chia seeds
- 1 cup unsweetened coconut milk
- 1/2 teaspoon vanilla extract
- 1 tablespoon sugar substitute
- 1/2 cup diced mango

Instructions:

1. Mix chia seeds, coconut milk, vanilla extract, and sugar substitute in a jar.
2. Refrigerate for at least 2 hours or overnight.
3. Layer the chia pudding with diced mango.
4. Enjoy a tropical delight guilt-free.

Nutrition Information:

- Calories: 120
- Protein: 3g
- Carbohydrates: 14g
- Fat: 6g

- Fiber: 8g
- Sugar: 4g
- Portion Size: 1/2 cup

Baked Apples with Cinnamon and Walnuts

Ingredients:

- 2 apples, cored and halved
- 1 teaspoon cinnamon
- 1/4 cup chopped walnuts
- 1 tablespoon sugar substitute
- 1/4 cup water

Instructions:

1. Preheat the oven to 375°F (190°C).
2. Place apples in a baking dish, sprinkle with cinnamon, walnuts, and sugar substitute.
3. Pour water into the dish.
4. Bake for 25-30 minutes until apples are tender.
5. Serve warm, and savor the natural sweetness.

Nutrition Information:

- Calories: 90
- Protein: 1g
- Carbohydrates: 15g
- Fat: 4g
- Fiber: 4g
- Sugar: 10g
- Portion Size: 1/2 baked apple

Pumpkin Pie Smoothie

Ingredients:

- 1/2 cup canned pumpkin puree
- 1/2 banana
- 1/2 cup unsweetened almond milk
- 1/2 teaspoon pumpkin pie spice
- 1 tablespoon sugar substitute
- Ice cubes

Instructions:

1. Blend pumpkin puree, banana, almond milk, pumpkin pie spice, and sugar substitute until smooth.

2. Add ice cubes and blend again for a refreshing smoothie.

3. Pour into a glass and sprinkle a dash of pumpkin spice on top.

Nutrition Information:

- Calories: 80
- Protein: 2g
- Carbohydrates: 15g
- Fat: 2g
- Fiber: 5g
- Sugar: 6g
- Portion Size: 1 cup

Lemon Poppy Seed Cake with Greek Yogurt Glaze

Ingredients:

- 1 cup almond flour
- 1/4 cup coconut flour
- 1 teaspoon baking powder
- 1/4 teaspoon salt
- 1/4 cup poppy seeds

- 1/4 cup lemon juice
- 1/4 cup sugar substitute
- 1/4 cup melted coconut oil
- 3 large eggs
- 1/2 cup Greek yogurt

Instructions:

1. Preheat the oven to 350°F (175°C) and grease a cake pan.
2. In a bowl, mix almond flour, coconut flour, baking powder, salt, and poppy seeds.
3. In another bowl, whisk lemon juice, sugar substitute, melted coconut oil, eggs, and Greek yogurt.
4. Combine wet and dry ingredients, then pour into the prepared pan.
5. Bake for 25-30 minutes until a toothpick comes out clean.

Nutrition Information:

- Calories: 160
- Protein: 5g
- Carbohydrates: 10g

- Fat: 12g
- Fiber: 3g
- Sugar: 2g
- Portion Size: 1 slice

Dark Chocolate-Dipped Strawberries

Ingredients:

- 1 cup dark chocolate chips (70% cocoa or higher)
- 1 pint fresh strawberries, washed and dried

Instructions:

1. Melt dark chocolate chips in a heatproof bowl over simmering water.
2. Dip each strawberry into the melted chocolate, coating them halfway.
3. Place on parchment paper and refrigerate until the chocolate hardens.
4. Enjoy this simple and elegant treat.

Nutrition Information:

- Calories: 50
- Protein: 1g

- Carbohydrates: 7g

- Fat: 3g

- Fiber: 2g

- Sugar: 4g

- Portion Size: 2 strawberries

Pistachio and Cranberry Energy Bites

Ingredients:

- 1 cup shelled pistachios

- 1/2 cup dried cranberries

- 1/4 cup almond butter

- 1/4 cup rolled oats

- 1 tablespoon chia seeds

- 1 teaspoon vanilla extract

- 1/4 cup sugar substitute

Instructions:

1. In a food processor, pulse pistachios until finely chopped.

2. Add cranberries, almond butter, oats, chia seeds, vanilla extract, and sugar substitute. Blend until mixture comes together.

3. Roll into bite-sized balls and refrigerate for at least 1 hour.

4. Energize yourself with these nutrient-packed bites.

Nutrition Information:

- Calories: 80
- Protein: 3g
- Carbohydrates: 7g
- Fat: 5g
- Fiber: 2g
- Sugar: 3g
- Portion Size: 2 bites

Raspberry and Almond Oat Bars

Ingredients:

- 1 cup rolled oats
- 1/2 cup almond flour
- 1/4 cup coconut oil, melted
- 1/4 cup sugar substitute

- 1/2 cup raspberry jam (no added sugar)
- 1/4 cup sliced almonds

Instructions:

1. Preheat the oven to 350°F (175°C) and line a baking pan with parchment paper.
2. In a bowl, combine rolled oats, almond flour, melted coconut oil, and sugar substitute.
3. Press half of the mixture into the bottom of the prepared pan.
4. Spread raspberry jam evenly over the oat layer.
5. Sprinkle the remaining oat mixture and sliced almonds on top.
6. Bake for 20-25 minutes or until the edges are golden brown.
7. Allow to cool before cutting into bars.

Nutrition Information:

- Calories: 120
- Protein: 3g
- Carbohydrates: 15g
- Fat: 6g

- Fiber: 2g
- Sugar: 5g
- Portion Size: 1 bar

Mango and Lime Frozen Yogurt

Ingredients:

- 2 cups frozen mango chunks
- 1 cup plain Greek yogurt
- 1 tablespoon lime zest
- 2 tablespoons lime juice
- 2 tablespoons honey or sugar substitute

Instructions:

1. Blend frozen mango chunks, Greek yogurt, lime zest, lime juice, and honey (or sugar substitute) until smooth.
2. Transfer the mixture into a shallow dish.
3. Freeze for at least 4 hours, stirring every hour.
4. Scoop into bowls and enjoy this tropical frozen delight.

Nutrition Information:

- Calories: 100
- Protein: 5g
- Carbohydrates: 20g
- Fat: 1g
- Fiber: 2g
- Sugar: 15g
- Portion Size: 1/2 cup

Vanilla Bean Panna Cotta with Berries

Ingredients:

- 2 cups unsweetened almond milk
- 1 tablespoon gelatin powder
- 1/4 cup sugar substitute
- 1 vanilla bean, seeds scraped
- Mixed berries for topping

Instructions:

1. In a saucepan, heat almond milk until warm but not boiling.

2. Sprinkle gelatin over almond milk and whisk until dissolved.

3. Add sugar substitute and vanilla bean seeds. Continue stirring until well combined.

4. Pour into ramekins and refrigerate for at least 4 hours or until set.

5. Top with mixed berries before serving.

Nutrition Information:

- Calories: 60
- Protein: 3g
- Carbohydrates: 2g
- Fat: 5g
- Fiber: 1g
- Sugar: 1g
- Portion Size: 1/2 cup

Peach and Almond Crisp

Ingredients:

- 4 cups sliced peaches
- 1 tablespoon lemon juice
- 1/4 cup sugar substitute

- 1/2 cup almond flour
- 1/4 cup rolled oats
- 1/4 cup sliced almonds
- 2 tablespoons coconut oil, melted

Instructions:

1. Preheat the oven to 350°F (175°C) and grease a baking dish.
2. Toss sliced peaches with lemon juice and sugar substitute. Place in the prepared dish.
3. In a bowl, combine almond flour, rolled oats, sliced almonds, and melted coconut oil.
4. Sprinkle the almond mixture over the peaches.
5. Bake for 30-35 minutes or until the top is golden brown.

Nutrition Information:

- Calories: 150
- Protein: 4g
- Carbohydrates: 20g
- Fat: 8g
- Fiber: 4g

- Sugar: 12g
- Portion Size: 1/2 cup

Carrot Cake Bites with Cream Cheese Frosting

Ingredients:

- 1 cup shredded carrots
- 1/2 cup almond flour
- 1/4 cup shredded coconut
- 1/4 cup chopped walnuts
- 1/4 cup dates, pitted
- 1/2 teaspoon cinnamon
- Cream cheese frosting (optional)

Instructions:

1. In a food processor, blend shredded carrots, almond flour, shredded coconut, chopped walnuts, dates, and cinnamon until a dough forms.
2. Roll the mixture into bite-sized balls.
3. If desired, drizzle with a small amount of cream cheese frosting.

Nutrition Information:

- Calories: 80
- Protein: 2g
- Carbohydrates: 10g
- Fat: 4g
- Fiber: 3g
- Sugar: 6g
- Portion Size: 2 bites

Banana and Walnut Bread Pudding

Ingredients:

- 3 ripe bananas, mashed
- 1/2 cup chopped walnuts
- 4 cups whole grain bread, cubed
- 2 cups unsweetened almond milk
- 3 large eggs
- 1/4 cup sugar substitute
- 1 teaspoon vanilla extract

Instructions:

1. Preheat the oven to 350°F (175°C) and grease a baking dish.

2. In a bowl, combine mashed bananas, chopped walnuts, and cubed bread.

3. In another bowl, whisk together almond milk, eggs, sugar substitute, and vanilla extract.

4. Pour the wet mixture over the bread mixture and let it sit for 10 minutes.

5. Bake for 30-35 minutes or until the top is golden brown.

Nutrition Information:
- Calories: 120
- Protein: 4g
- Carbohydrates: 15g
- Fat: 5g
- Fiber: 3g
- Sugar: 6g
- Portion Size: 1/2 cup

Chapter 7: Smoothies

In this Chapter, we delve into the vibrant world of smoothies, offering not just delicious concoctions but a blend of nutrients tailored to boost your well-being. Let's embark on a smoothie adventure that transcends the ordinary.

Green Goddess Detox Smoothie

Ingredients:

- 1 cup kale, stemmed and chopped
- 1/2 cucumber, peeled and sliced
- 1 green apple, cored and chopped
- 1/2 lemon, juiced
- 1 cup coconut water
- Ice cubes (optional)

Instructions:

1. Blend all ingredients until smooth.
2. Pour into a glass and enjoy!

Nutrition Information:

- Calories: 120

- Protein: 3g

- Carbohydrates: 28g

- Fat: 1g

- Fiber: 5g

- Sugar: 15g

- Portion size: 1 serving

Berry Blast Antioxidant Smoothie

Ingredients:

- 1 cup mixed berries (strawberries, blueberries, raspberries)

- 1/2 banana

- 1/2 cup Greek yogurt

- 1 tablespoon chia seeds

- 1 cup almond milk

- Ice cubes (optional)

Instructions:

1. Blend all ingredients until smooth.

2. Pour into a glass and savor the berry goodness!

Nutrition Information:

- Calories: 150
- Protein: 7g
- Carbohydrates: 25g
- Fat: 3g
- Fiber: 8g
- Sugar: 12g
- Portion size: 1 serving

Tropical Turmeric Smoothie

Ingredients:

- 1 cup mango, diced
- 1/2 cup pineapple chunks
- 1 teaspoon turmeric powder
- 1 tablespoon flaxseeds
- 1 cup coconut water
- Ice cubes (optional)

Instructions:

1. Blend all ingredients until smooth.
2. Pour into a glass and transport yourself to the tropics!

Nutrition Information:

- Calories: 140
- Protein: 4g
- Carbohydrates: 30g
- Fat: 2g
- Fiber: 6g
- Sugar: 18g
- Portion size: 1 serving

Spinach and Pineapple Power Smoothie

Ingredients:

- 2 cups fresh spinach
- 1 cup pineapple chunks
- 1/2 banana
- 1 tablespoon hemp seeds
- 1 cup water
- Ice cubes (optional)

Instructions:

1. Blend all ingredients until smooth.
2. Pour into a glass and feel the power!

Nutrition Information:

- Calories: 130
- Protein: 5g
- Carbohydrates: 28g
- Fat: 2g
- Fiber: 5g
- Sugar: 15g
- Portion size: 1 serving

Chocolate Almond Butter Protein Smoothie

Ingredients:

- 1 cup almond milk
- 1 tablespoon almond butter
- 1 scoop chocolate protein powder
- 1/2 banana
- 1 tablespoon cacao nibs
- Ice cubes (optional)

Instructions:

1. Blend all ingredients until smooth.
2. Pour into a glass and indulge guilt-free!

Nutrition Information:

- Calories: 180
- Protein: 20g
- Carbohydrates: 15g
- Fat: 8g
- Fiber: 4g
- Sugar: 6g
- Portion size: 1 serving

Avocado and Kale Energy Boost Smoothie

Ingredients:

- 1/2 avocado
- 1 cup kale, stemmed and chopped
- 1/2 cup mango chunks
- 1 tablespoon chia seeds
- 1 cup coconut water
- Ice cubes (optional)

Instructions:

1. Blend all ingredients until smooth.
2. Pour into a glass and experience an energy boost!

Nutrition Information:

- Calories: 160
- Protein: 5g
- Carbohydrates: 24g
- Fat: 8g
- Fiber: 7g
- Sugar: 12g
- Portion size: 1 serving

Citrus Burst Immune Booster Smoothie

Ingredients:

- 1 orange, peeled and segmented
- 1/2 cup pineapple chunks
- 1/2 lemon, juiced
- 1 tablespoon ginger, grated
- 1 cup water
- Ice cubes (optional)

Instructions:

1. Blend all ingredients until smooth.

2. Pour into a glass and give your immune system a
   boost!

Nutrition Information:

- Calories: 110
- Protein: 2g
- Carbohydrates: 28g
- Fat: 1g
- Fiber: 4g
- Sugar: 18g
- Portion size: 1 serving

Beet and Berry Antioxidant Smoothie

Ingredients:

- 1/2 cup cooked beets, diced
- 1/2 cup mixed berries (strawberries, blueberries)
- 1/2 banana
- 1 tablespoon flaxseeds
- 1 cup almond milk
- Ice cubes (optional)

Instructions:

1. Blend all ingredients until smooth.
2. Pour into a glass and revel in the antioxidant goodness!

Nutrition Information:

- Calories: 140
- Protein: 4g
- Carbohydrates: 25g
- Fat: 3g
- Fiber: 8g
- Sugar: 12g
- Portion size: 1 serving

Cucumber Mint Refreshing Smoothie

Ingredients:

- 1 cucumber, peeled and sliced
- 1/2 cup fresh mint leaves
- 1/2 green apple, cored and chopped
- 1 tablespoon chia seeds
- 1 cup coconut water
- Ice cubes (optional)

Instructions:

1. Blend all ingredients until smooth.

2. Pour into a glass and refresh your senses!

Nutrition Information:

- Calories: 90

- Protein: 2g

- Carbohydrates: 20g

- Fat: 1g

- Fiber: 5g

- Sugar: 10g

- Portion size: 1 serving

Pomegranate and Blueberry Delight Smoothie

Ingredients:

- 1/2 cup pomegranate seeds

- 1/2 cup blueberries

- 1/2 banana

- 1 tablespoon hemp seeds

- 1 cup almond milk

- Ice cubes (optional)

Instructions:

1. Blend all ingredients until smooth.
2. Pour into a glass and savor the delightful blend!

Nutrition Information:

- Calories: 130
- Protein: 5g
- Carbohydrates: 25g
- Fat: 3g
- Fiber: 6g
- Sugar: 15g
- Portion size: 1 serving

Mango Tango Anti-Inflammatory Smoothie

Ingredients:

- 1 cup mango chunks
- 1/2 teaspoon turmeric powder
- 1/2 teaspoon ginger, grated
- 1 tablespoon flaxseeds
- 1 cup coconut water
- Ice cubes (optional)

Instructions:

1. Blend all ingredients until smooth.
2. Pour into a glass and dance with the anti-inflammatory goodness!

Nutrition Information:

- Calories: 150
- Protein: 3g
- Carbohydrates: 30g
- Fat: 2g
- Fiber: 5g
- Sugar: 18g
- Portion size: 1 serving

Coffee and Almond Milk Smoothie

Ingredients:

- 1 cup brewed coffee, cooled
- 1/2 cup almond milk
- 1/2 banana
- 1 tablespoon almond butter
- 1 teaspoon vanilla extract
- Ice cubes (optional)

Instructions:

1. Blend all ingredients until smooth.
2. Pour into a glass and enjoy a caffeinated pick-me-up!

Nutrition Information:

- Calories: 80
- Protein: 2g
- Carbohydrates: 15g
- Fat: 4g
- Fiber: 3g
- Sugar: 8g
- Portion size: 1 serving

Mixed Berry and Spinach Green Smoothie

Ingredients:

- 1 cup mixed berries (strawberries, blueberries, raspberries)
- 1 cup fresh spinach
- 1/2 banana
- 1 tablespoon chia seeds
- 1 cup water

- Ice cubes (optional)

Instructions:

1. Blend all ingredients until smooth.
2. Pour into a glass and relish the green goodness!

Nutrition Information:

- Calories: 120
- Protein: 4g
- Carbohydrates: 25g
- Fat: 3g
- Fiber: 8g
- Sugar: 12g
- Portion size: 1 serving

Peanut Butter Banana Protein Smoothie

Ingredients:

- 1/2 banana
- 1 tablespoon peanut butter
- 1 scoop vanilla protein powder
- 1 cup almond milk

- 1 tablespoon flaxseeds

- Ice cubes (optional)

Instructions:

1. Blend all ingredients until smooth.

2. Pour into a glass and relish the protein-packed delight!

Nutrition Information:

- Calories: 180

- Protein: 20g

- Carbohydrates: 15g

- Fat: 8g

- Fiber: 4g

- Sugar: 6g

- Portion size: 1 serving

Cherry Almond Recovery Smoothie

Ingredients:

- 1/2 cup cherries, pitted

- 1/4 cup almonds

- 1/2 cup Greek yogurt

- 1 tablespoon honey
- 1 cup water
- Ice cubes (optional)

Instructions:

1. Blend all ingredients until smooth.
2. Pour into a glass and enjoy a delicious recovery treat!

Nutrition Information:

- Calories: 200
- Protein: 10g
- Carbohydrates: 20g
- Fat: 10g
- Fiber: 3g
- Sugar: 15g
- Portion size: 1 serving

CONCLUSION

Throughout the chapters, we've explored the intricacies of diabetic nutrition, delving into the benefits of a vegetarian diet. The 30-day meal plan serves as a roadmap, guiding readers through a diverse array of breakfasts, lunches, dinners, snacks, desserts, and smoothies. Each recipe is a celebration of taste and health, meticulously designed to tantalize taste buds while promoting stable blood sugar levels.

The breakfast selections welcome each day with a burst of energy, from the indulgent Sweet Potato Hash with Poached Eggs to the refreshing Mango Lime Smoothie. Our lunch recipes offer a symphony of flavors, introducing inventive dishes like the Thai Basil Tofu Stir-Fry and the Mediterranean Stuffed Portobello Mushrooms. As the day winds down, dinner options such as the Butternut Squash and Sage Risotto or the Ratatouille with Herbed Quinoa bring a comforting conclusion.

For those in-between moments, the snacks and appetizers provide satisfying bites, from the Guacamole with Veggie Sticks to the Mini Caprese Salad Skewers. Desserts become a guilt-free pleasure with creations like the Chocolate Avocado Mousse and the Almond Flour Blueberry Muffins, proving that sweetness and health can coexist. Finally, our smoothie recipes serve as vibrant elixirs, combining taste and nutrition in each refreshing sip.

This cookbook extends beyond a mere collection of recipes; it's an invitation to embrace a lifestyle where health and culinary delight intertwine. It empowers beginners to navigate the world of vegetarian diabetic cooking with confidence, demonstrating that nourishing the body can be a joyous and flavorful experience. May these recipes not only inspire delicious meals but also foster a newfound appreciation for the art of crafting wholesome, diabetic-friendly dishes. Here's to a journey of culinary exploration and well-being!

* 9 7 9 8 8 7 8 5 6 3 4 2 0 *